MEAL PREP COOKBOOK

Simple, easy, quick and delicious daily
recipes to prepare your favorite
restaurant dishes at home

Table of Contents

Introduction

Why is this Meal Prep Cookbook release so important? Because at MEAL PREP, we believe in the power of preparing today's foods with the assurance that you'll always have healthy options to get the body and mind ready for tomorrow. This cookbook is full of easy recipes that will save you money and help you achieve your fitness goals.

In recent years, Meal Prep has become an emerging trend as people realize the benefits of spending time preparing meals in advance. Convenience, cost-effectiveness, and time-saving are the main factors contributing to the growing popularity of meal prep. If you are a busy working professional, meal prep will help you cut down on the money and time you spend on buying take-outs from the office cafeteria. It will also help you stay away from junk food and better control your caloric intake. Preparing a few portions of your favorite meals can help you save money and feel energetic enough to make it through the long and busy work schedule and daily responsibilities.

The most significant advantage of prepping your own meals is the chance to personalize your meals. This factor makes prepping meals more enjoyable and exciting. Individuals used to buy prepared meals from their local grocery stores and take their meals to work. It cost money and took up most of their time only to have it eaten in front of them while they are sitting at their desks all day.

While the benefits of meal prep can be split into two main categories: financial and health, it saves lots of your finances in the long run by reaping the benefits of cheaper food. You will also enjoy healthier eating because you already chose what and how much to eat. Not to mention, meal prep is an excellent way to stay consistent with your goals and objectives. For anyone who wants to lose weight, for example, the key to long-term success is consistency. To succeed with weight loss, you must stay in control of your diet. If you are going about it the right way and planning ahead, you will lose weight much easier than you ever thought possible.

It also allows you to eat healthy throughout the week without worrying about finding time to shop or cook. This meal prep cookbook includes a wide range of recipes so that you can use this book for multiple purposes. You can use these recipes for meal prepping, as well as making them from scratch for your family and friends.

How to Meal Prep?

There are different ways on how you can meal prep if you're a beginner in this journey. Some of them are the following:

Make-Ahead Meals

Prepare for the week ahead and freeze the meals that you plan to cook every week. This kind of meal preparation is easy and saves time in the summer. Using freezer containers is a great way to preserve food for future use. The frozen meals taste great and have fewer ingredients. You will also save your wallet on fresh groceries.

Batch Cooking

This meal prep method involves preparing multiple recipes at a time and cooking them all together. It is an excellent way to prepare several meals fast. This method's advantage is that it is economical since you can prepare large portions of food in one go.

Individually Portioned Meals

Prepare food individually and make sure they will be ready fast. This method is perfect for a week filled with celebrations. You can prepare each meal individually in the evening and enjoy the benefits of eating right out of the containers.

Ready-To-Cook Ingredients

If you're a busy person who does not have much time to cook in the morning, shopping for ready-to-cook ingredients will do. Buying and preparing fresh ingredients ahead of time will help you save time in the busy mornings. But make sure to eat fresh meals. As soon as the ingredients are bought, they will also spoil if not eaten straight away. Therefore, you need to plan your meals ahead of time to make sure you will use them before they get stale.

Now that you know the basics and advantages of meal prepping, it's time to get down to the most awaited 500 meal prep recipes with the 30-day meal plan by the end of it. We hope you'll enjoy the wide range of meals but make sure to make them in your own way. If you are a vegan, don't add meat to your recipes. If you are a vegetarian, add some meat to the recipe. Most importantly, don't fear to play around with your recipes! Happy meal prepping.

Lemon Cheesecake Mousse

Preparation time: 15 minutes
Cooking time: 0 minutes
Servings: 6
Ingredients:

- 8 ounces cream cheese, softened
- Juice from 2 large lemons, about 1/4 cup
- 1 cup coconut cream
- 1/2 teaspoon liquid stevia
- 1/4 teaspoon lemon extract
- 1/8 teaspoon salt

Directions:

1. Beat cream cheese in your medium mixing bowl. Add lemon juice and beat until smooth. Add remaining ingredients and beat until just combined. Split into six glass jars with lids. Store in the refrigerator.

Nutrition:
Calories: 201
Fat: 20 g
Protein: 3 g
Carbohydrates: 2.5 g

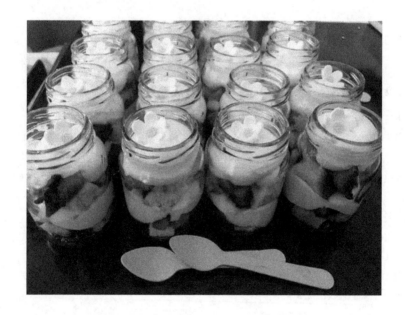

Cashew Butter Mousse

Preparation time: 15 minutes
Cooking time: 0 minutes
Servings: 6
Ingredients:

- 8 ounces cream cheese, softened
- 1/4 cup no-sugar-added creamy cashew butter
- 10 drops liquid stevia
- 1 teaspoon vanilla extract
- 1 cup heavy whipping cream, chilled

Directions:

1. Combine all ingredients except whipping cream in a medium mixing bowl and beat until smooth. Set aside.
2. Beat the whipping cream until stiff peaks in a separate medium bowl. Fold whipped cream into the cashew butter mixture and beat 1 minute or until a fluffy mousse form.
3. Divide mousse into six equal portions and transfer to glass jars with lids. Store in the refrigerator.

Nutrition:
Calories: 274
Fat: 28 g
Protein: 3 g
Carbohydrates: 3 g

Mint Chocolate Brownies

Preparation time: 15 minutes
Cooking time: 30 minutes
Servings: 6
Ingredients:

- 1/2 cup chocolate chips (sweetened with stevia)
- 1/2 cup grass-fed butter
- 3 large eggs
- 1/4 cup granulated erythritol
- 1/2 teaspoon peppermint extract

Directions:

1. Preheat oven to 350°F. Grease an 8" × 8" baking dish. Mix chocolate chips plus butter in a small saucepan. Heat over low heat until melted. Remove from heat immediately.
2. Combine remaining fixings in a medium mixing bowl and beat until frothy. Pour chocolate mixture into the egg mixture and beat until fully incorporated.
3. Pour batter into your prepared baking dish, then bake 30 minutes or until a toothpick inserted in the center comes out clean.
4. Allow to cool completely and cut into six equal slices. Store each piece in an airtight container or snack bag—store at room temperature.

Nutrition:
Calories: 178
Fat: 18 g
Protein: 3 g
Carbohydrates: 9g

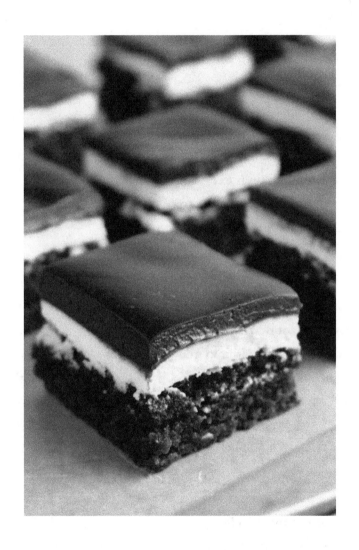

Pumpkin Pie Bites

Preparation time: 15 minutes
Cooking time: 0 minutes
Servings: 12
Ingredients:

- 21/2 cups unsweetened, shredded coconut
- 1/2 cup coconut oil
- 1/2 teaspoon liquid stevia
- 1/4 teaspoon coarse salt
- 1/4 cup collagen powder
- 3/4 cup pumpkin purée, room temperature
- 1 tablespoon pumpkin pie spice
- 1/2 teaspoon vanilla extract

Directions:

1. Prepare 12 cups of a mini muffin tin with cupcake liners. Combine shredded coconut, coconut oil, stevia, and salt in the bowl of a food processor.
2. Process on high within 5 minutes or until a smooth "butter" form. You need to stop the food processor and scrape the sides of the bowl a few times.
3. Remove 1/4 cup of coconut mixture and pour evenly into prepared muffin cups. Add remaining ingredients to coconut mixture in the food processor and blend until smooth.
4. Scoop pumpkin mixture onto coconut mixture in muffin tins and spread out evenly.
5. Place the muffin tin in your freezer for 1 hour or until set. Put two pumpkin bites in separate snack bags and store them in the freezer until ready to eat.

Nutrition:

Calories: 280
Fat: 29 g
Protein: 1 g
Carbohydrates: 6 g

Chocolate Pudding

Preparation time: 15 minutes
Cooking time: 0 minutes
Servings: 6
Ingredients:

- 3 cups full-fat coconut milk
- 1/3 cup unsweetened cacao powder
- 1/4 cup granulated erythritol
- 2 teaspoons instant coffee
- 1 teaspoon vanilla extract
- 3 tablespoons grass-fed gelatin
- 1/3 cup water

Directions:

1. Combine coconut milk, cacao powder, erythritol, coffee, and vanilla extract in a small saucepan. Mix with a whisk over medium heat until combined and frothy.
2. In a small bowl, mix gelatin and water. Add to saucepan and whisk until gelatin is fully dissolved.
3. Transfer pudding mixture evenly to six glass jars with lids and refrigerate until set, about 1 hour. Put in the fridge until the time you're ready to eat it.

Nutrition:
Calories: 285
Fat: 24 g
Protein: 14 g
Carbohydrates: 16 g

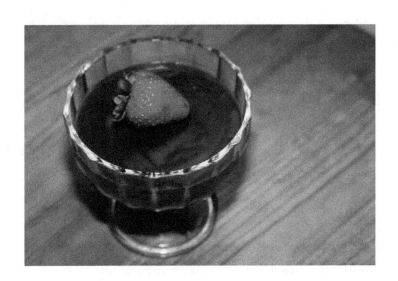

Cinnamon Bites

Preparation time: 15 minutes
Cooking time: 0 minutes
Servings: 12
Ingredients:

- 1/2 cup no-sugar-added sunflower seed butter
- 2 teaspoons cinnamon, divided
- 3 tablespoons coconut flour
- 3 tablespoons almond milk
- 1/4 cup plus 3 tablespoons erythritol, divided
- 1/2 teaspoon vanilla extract
- 1/4 teaspoon salt

Directions:

1. Combine sunflower seed butter, 1 teaspoon cinnamon, coconut flour, almond milk, 1/4 cup erythritol, vanilla extract, and salt in a medium bowl. Mix until incorporated.
2. Combine the remaining cinnamon and erythritol in a separate small bowl. Set aside. Roll dough into 1" round balls. Drop each ball into cinnamon and erythritol mixture and toss to coat.
3. Move it to a baking sheet lined using parchment paper and chill in the refrigerator for 2 hours. Once cooled, place two cinnamon bites in each of six snack baggies and store them in the refrigerator until ready to eat.

Nutrition:
Calories: 141
Fat: 11 g
Protein: 5.5 g
Carbohydrates: 22 g

Pistachio Fudge

Preparation time: 15 minutes
Cooking time: 0 minutes
Servings: 12
Ingredients:

- 9 tablespoons grass-fed butter, softened
- 4 ounces cream cheese, softened
- 3 tablespoons cacao powder
- 2 tablespoons granulated erythritol
- 1 teaspoon vanilla extract
- 1/2 cup shelled pistachio pieces

Directions:

1. Beat butter plus cream cheese until smooth in a medium mixing bowl. Add cacao powder, erythritol, and vanilla extract and stir to combine. Fold in pistachio pieces.
2. Press evenly into an 8" × 8" baking dish lined with parchment paper. Put in your refrigerator and allow to chill 1 hour.
3. Remove and cut into twelve equal-sized pieces. Put each piece in a snack bag and store it in the refrigerator until ready to eat.

Nutrition:
Calories: 141
Fat: 14 g
Protein: 2 g
Carbohydrates: 5 g

Vanilla Mascarpone Parfait

Preparation time: 15 minutes
Cooking time: 0 minutes
Servings: 6
Ingredients:

- 1 cup mascarpone cheese
- 1 cup coconut cream
- 3/4 teaspoon liquid stevia
- 1/2 teaspoon vanilla extract
- 3/4 cup sliced strawberries

Directions:

1. Combine mascarpone, coconut cream, stevia, and vanilla extract in a medium mixing bowl. Beat until peaks start to form, about 2 minutes.
2. Place 1 tablespoon strawberries in the bottom of each of six glass jars with lids—top strawberries with equal amounts of the mascarpone mixture. Add 1 tablespoon strawberries to the top of each jar. Cover and refrigerate until ready to eat.

Nutrition:
Calories: 213
Fat: 21 g
Protein: 3 g
Carbohydrates: 4g

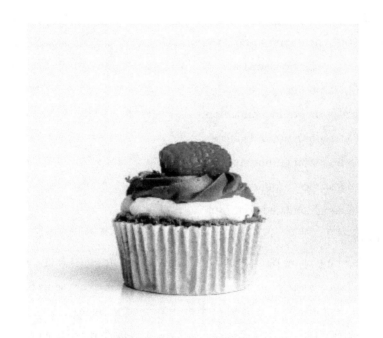

Pumpkin Spice Pudding

Preparation time: 15 minutes
Cooking time: 0 minutes
Servings: 6
Ingredients:

- 1/4 cup water
- 1 tablespoon grass-fed gelatin
- 1 (14-ounce) can pumpkin purée
- 1 (14-ounce) can full-fat coconut milk
- 2 teaspoons vanilla extract
- 1/4 teaspoon salt
- 1 teaspoon ground cinnamon
- 1/4 teaspoon ground ginger
- 1/8 teaspoon ground nutmeg
- 1/8 teaspoon ground cloves
- 1/4 cup granulated erythritol

Directions:

1. Combine water plus gelatin in a small bowl. Stir to get rid of clumps and set aside. Combine remaining fixings in a medium saucepan and stir over low heat until smooth and warmed through.
2. Remove from heat and stir in prepared gelatin. Transfer pudding mixture to six glass jars with lids and place in the refrigerator until set, about 1 hour. Store in refrigerator until ready to eat.

Nutrition:
Calories: 172
Fat: 14 g
Protein: 6 g
Carbohydrates: 15g

Sunflower Butter Chocolate Bars

Preparation time: 15 minutes
Cooking time: 5 minutes
Servings: 12
Ingredients:

- 11/4 cup almond flour
- 6 ounces grass-fed butter
- 1/3 cup powdered erythritol
- 3/4 cup no-sugar-added sunflower seed butter
- 3/4 teaspoon vanilla extract
- 3/4 cup chocolate chips (sweetened with stevia)

Directions:

1. Combine all ingredients except chocolate chips in a medium bowl and beat until smooth. Press into an 8" × 8" baking dish lined with parchment paper.
2. Heat-up the chocolate chips in a small saucepan over low heat. Stir constantly until chocolate is melted. Remove from heat and pour onto sunflower seed butter mixture immediately.
3. Spread chocolate out evenly on top. Allow chilling in the refrigerator for 2 hours or until hardened.
4. Once hardened, remove from refrigerator and cut into twelve equal-sized bars. Transfer bars to snack bags and store in the refrigerator until ready to eat.

Nutrition:
Calories: 230
Fat: 17 g
Protein: 3 g
Carbohydrates: 22 g

Peanut Butter Cookies

Preparation time: 15 minutes
Cooking time: 12 minutes
Servings: 12 cookies
Ingredients:

- 1 cup granulated erythritol
- 1 cup no-sugar-added peanut butter
- 1 large egg

Directions:

1. Preheat oven to 350°F. Line a baking sheet with parchment paper. Combine fixings in a medium mixing bowl and beat until dough forms.
2. Using your hands, form 1" balls with the dough and place balls on the prepared baking sheet. Create a crisscross pattern in the top of each dough ball using a fork.
3. Bake 12 minutes or until cookies are slightly browned. Remove from oven and allow to cool. Once cooled, put two cookies into each of six snack baggies. Store at room temperature.

Nutrition:
Calories: 267
Fat: 22 g
Protein: 10 g
Carbohydrates: 41 g

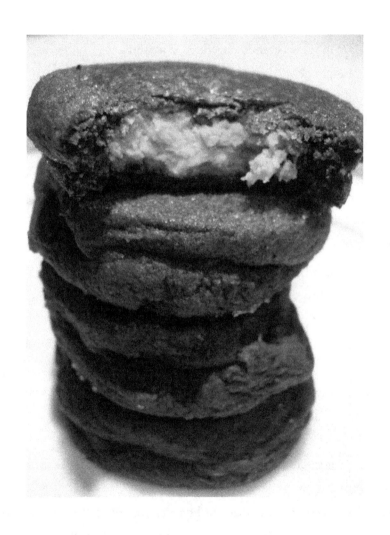

Chocolate Coconut Clusters

Preparation time: 15 minutes
Cooking time: 15 minutes
Servings: 12
Ingredients:

- 2/3 cup unsweetened shredded coconut
- 1/4 cup coconut cream
- 2 tablespoons unsalted grass-fed butter
- 3 tablespoons cacao powder
- 3 tablespoons erythritol
- 1/8 teaspoon salt
- 1/4 cup no-sugar-added sunflower seed butter

Directions:

1. Preheat oven to 350°F. Put shredded coconut out in a single layer on a baking sheet. Bake 5 minutes or until starting to slightly brown, flipping coconut over once during baking. Remove from oven and set aside.
2. Combine coconut cream, butter, cacao powder, erythritol, and salt in a small saucepan over medium heat. Stir and then bring to a simmer. Remove from heat and stir in sunflower seed butter until smooth.
3. Fold toasted coconut flakes into cacao mixture until incorporated. Drop by spoonful onto your baking sheet lined with parchment paper.
4. Place in the refrigerator until hardened, about 1 hour. Transfer clusters to an airtight container or individual snack bags and stores them in the refrigerator until ready to eat.

Nutrition:
Calories: 77

Fat: 7 g
Protein: 1.5 g
Carbohydrates: 6 g

Peanut Butter Fudge

Preparation time: 15 minutes
Cooking time: 10 minutes
Servings: 12
Ingredients:

- 1 cup no-sugar-added creamy peanut butter
- 1 cup plus 3 tablespoons coconut oil, divided
- 1/4 cup coconut milk
- 2 teaspoons liquid stevia
- 1/2 teaspoon vanilla extract
- 1/4 cup unsweetened cacao powder
- 2 tablespoons granulated erythritol

Directions:

1. Line an 8" × 8" baking pan using parchment paper. Place peanut butter and 1 cup coconut oil into a small saucepan over low heat. Stir until combined. Add coconut milk, stevia, and vanilla extract and stir until smooth.
2. Pour mixture into prepared baking dish. Put remaining coconut oil, cacao powder, and erythritol in a small saucepan and stir over low heat until combined—drizzle cacao mixture over peanut butter mixture.
3. Drag a toothpick through the mixture to create a swirl pattern. Refrigerate until hardened, about 2 hours.
4. Once the fudge has hardened, cut into twelve equal-sized squares and transfer each square to a snack bag or airtight container. Put in the fridge until the time you're ready to eat it.

Nutrition:
Calories: 331
Fat: 33 g

Protein: 5 g
Carbohydrates: 7 g

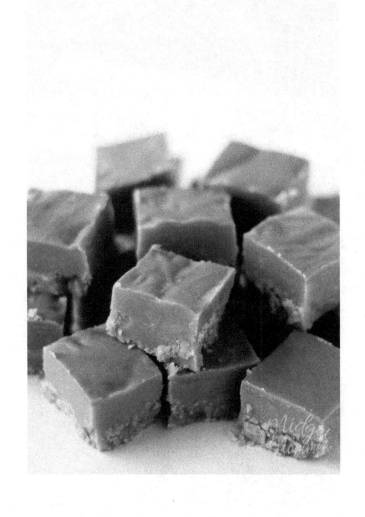

Snickerdoodle Cupcakes

Preparation time: 15 minutes
Cooking time: 20-25 minutes
Servings: 12
Ingredients:

- 1 cup unsalted grass-fed butter, softened
- 1/2 cup granulated erythritol
- 3 large eggs
- 2 teaspoons vanilla extract
- 1/4 cup heavy cream
- 3 tablespoons water
- 1/3 cup coconut flour
- 1 cup almond flour
- 1 teaspoon baking powder
- 1/4 teaspoon salt
- 2 teaspoons cinnamon
- 1/2 teaspoon nutmeg
- 1/4 cup crushed walnuts

Directions:

1. Warm oven to 350°F. Prepare a lined 12-cup muffin pan with cupcake liners. Beat softened butter in a medium bowl until light and fluffy.
2. Add erythritol and continue beating until incorporated. Add eggs, vanilla, cream, and water and beat until smooth. Set aside.
3. Combine remaining ingredients except for walnuts in a separate medium bowl. Fold dry ingredients into wet ingredients and stir until just combined. Fold in walnuts.
4. Fill muffin wells evenly and bake 20–25 minutes or until the toothpick inserted in the center comes out clean.

5. Once cooled, transfer each cupcake to an airtight container or snack bag and store at room temperature.

Nutrition:
Calories: 234
Fat: 20 g
Protein: 4 g
Carbohydrates: 19 g

Pineapple Spice Sorbet

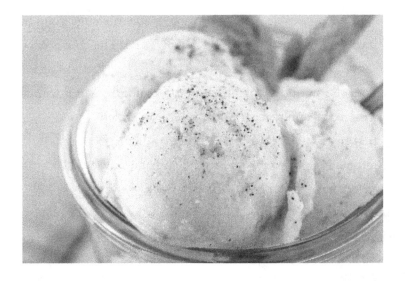

Preparation time: 15 minutes
Cooking time: 0 minutes
Servings: 4
Ingredients:

- 1 pineapple (peeled, cored, and chopped)
- 1 lime juice
- 1 piece of ginger (fresh and minced)
- 1/3 cup of coconut sugar
- 1/8 cup of basil leaves (fresh)

Directions:

1. Add the pineapple, lime juice, ginger, coconut sugar, and basil leaves to a blender. Blend on a high speed. The consistency should be smooth.
2. Pour the smoothie mixture into a container, cover it with an airtight lid, and place it in the freezer overnight.
3. Before serving, remove the sorbet container from the refrigerator, allow it to defrost slightly before serving. Store the sorbet in your freezer for up to a week.

Nutrition:
Calories: 145
Carbohydrates: 33g
Protein: 1.4g
Fat: 0.1g

Cherry Almond Brownies

Preparation time: 15 minutes
Cooking time: 45 minutes
Servings: 4
Ingredients:

- 1 cup of coconut sugar
- 1/3 cup of vegan butter
- 1/3 cup of glace' cherry
- 1/3 cup of ground almonds
- ½ cup of vegan dark chocolate
- ½ cup of flour (self-raising)
- 6 tbsp of water
- 2 tbsp of cocoa powder
- 2 tbsp of ground flaxseed
- 1 ½ tsp of vanilla extract
- 1/3 tsp of coffee
- ¼ tsp of baking powder

Directions:

1. Heat the oven to 330 degrees-Fahrenheit, and line a square tin with parchment paper. Combine the ground flaxseed with 6 tbsp of water in a bowl, and set it aside for 5 minutes.

2. Heat-up a small pan over medium heat, and melt the dark chocolate, coffee, and vegan butter in the pan. Put 3 tbsp of water into the pan. Once melted, remove from the heat.

3. Add the flour, cocoa, baking powder, almonds, and salt to a bowl. Whisk the ingredients to combine. Add the coconut sugar and melted chocolate-coffee mixture to the dry ingredients, and mix everything until you've reached a smooth consistency.

4. Mix vanilla extract, the flaxseed mixture, cherries, and flour mixture, stirring all the ingredients until well combined. The consistency should be very thick.

5. Spoon all of the batters into the tin. Bake the brownies for 40 minutes. Then, remove them from the oven, allowing them to cool down first before cutting them into squares.

6. Store the brownies in an airtight container between sheets of parchment paper for up to 3 days.

Nutrition:
Calories: 295
Carbohydrates: 34g
Protein: 4g
Fat: 15g

Raspberry Chia Pudding

Preparation time: 15 minutes
Cooking time: 0 minutes
Servings: 4
Ingredients:

- 2 cup of coconut milk
- peaches (sliced)
- 5 tbsp of chia seeds
- 4 tbsp of goji berries
- Raspberry glaze: 1 cup of raspberries, 4 tsp of agave, and 2 tsp of lemon juice

Directions:

1. Prepare 4 mason jars by dividing the chia seeds and coconut milk evenly between them. Stir the contents of each jar well, and leave it to soak for 5 to 6 minutes while stirring it each minute to ensure the seeds swell properly and don't stick to the jar.
2. Mix the raspberries, agave, plus lemon juice in a blender, and scoop 1 to 1 ½ spoon thereof into each mason jar.
3. Cover with a lid, and refrigerate the raspberry chia pudding in the refrigerator for up to 2 days. Serve with half of 1 sliced peach and 1 tbsp of goji berries per jar.

Nutrition:
Calories: 255
Carbohydrates: 25.4g
Protein: 8g
Fat: 10g

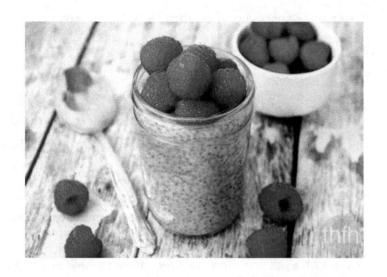

Sweet Tiffin

Preparation time: 15 minutes
Cooking time: 3 minutes
Servings: 4
Ingredients:

- 1 cup of dark chocolate (vegan)
- 2/3 cups of macadamia nuts
- 1/3 cup of dried cranberries
- 1/3 cup of coconut oil
- ¼ cup of pistachios
- 2 tbsp of maple syrup

Directions:

1. Spray a brownie tin with cooking spray. Layer the tin with a single sheet of parchment paper.
2. Add the chocolate and maple syrup to a microwaveable bowl, and microwave it for 30 seconds or until you reach a smooth consistency.
3. Crush the nuts into smaller pieces in a bowl. Add the cranberries and pistachios. Mix the ingredients to combine, and add the chocolate mixture to the bowl. Mix once more, then pour the mixture into the brownie tin.
4. Press the mixture with the back of a spoon to ensure it creates a flat, even layer. Refrigerate it within 2 hours before cutting it into squares, about 4-inches in length and width.
5. Place the brownies in an airtight container between parchment paper sheets and refrigerate it for up to 5 days.

Nutrition:
Calories: 130
Carbohydrates: 10g
Protein: 1.1g
Fat: 9g

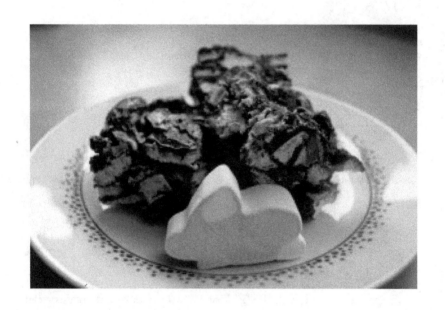

Banana Peanut Butter Muffins

Preparation time: 15 minutes
Cooking time: 20 minutes
Servings: 4
Ingredients:

- 1 cup of flour (self-raising)
- 1 cup of mayonnaise (egg-free)
- 2/3 cups of caster sugar
- 2 bananas (mashed)
- 2tbsp of vegan dark chocolate chips
- 1 tsp of bicarbonate soda
- 1 tsp of vanilla extract
- ¼ tsp of salt

Cupcake icing:

- 4 tbsp of vegan margarine
- 1 cup of icing sugar
- 2 tbsp of peanut butter
- 1 tbsp of almond milk

Directions:

1. Heat the oven to 360 degrees-Fahrenheit, and line a muffin tin with 12 muffin cups. Add the flour, caster sugar, bicarbonate soda, and salt to a bowl, and mix them.
2. Add the mayonnaise, vanilla extract, mashed bananas to another bowl, and mix the ingredients.
3. Add the wet fixings to the dry ingredients, and spoon the mixture into the muffin tin cups, dividing it evenly. Bake it for 20 minutes.
4. Remove the cupcakes, and sprinkle chocolate chips on top while they are still hot to melt.

5. Prepare the icing in another bowl by combining the icing sugar and vegan margarine with an electric mixer. Mix it for 2 to 3 minutes.

6. Once done, stir in the peanut butter, and spread the icing on top of the cupcakes. Store the cupcakes in a square glass container for 3 days.

Nutrition:
Calories: 300
Carbohydrates: 40g
Protein: 2.1g
Fat: 14g

Vegan Mince Pies

Preparation time: 15 minutes
Cooking time: 1 hour & 10 minutes
Servings: 4
Ingredients:

- 1 apple (peeled and grated)
- 1 cup of mixed dry fruit (no added sugar)
- 1 ½ cups of black cherries
- 1/3 cup of hazelnuts (roasted and chopped roughly)
- 2 tbsp of water
- 1 tsp of ginger
- 1 tsp of cinnamon
- ½ tsp of turmeric

Pastry:

- 1 ½ cups of flour
- ¾ cup of coconut oil
- 1 tbsp of icing sugar
- 2 tbsp of almond milk.

Directions:

1. Heat the oven to 360 degrees-Fahrenheit. Add the grated apple, dried fruit, half the black cherries, chopped hazelnuts, ginger, cinnamon, and turmeric to a casserole dish, mixing the ingredients.
2. Bake it in the oven within 35 minutes. Once done, set it aside to cool down.
3. Add the coconut oil and flour to a food processor. Pulse the mixture until it reaches a breadcrumb consistency. Add the icing sugar, and pulse once more to combine. Add 2 tbsp of water, and pulse again for the pastry to develop properly.

4. Put the dough on parchment paper, patting it into a round ball with your hands. Cover it in foil, then let it chill in the refrigerator for up to 30 minutes.

5. Once done, remove the pastry from the refrigerator and cut off 1/3 of the pastry, keeping it covered. Cut the remaining into 5 parts. Take each part and separately squeeze it with your hands.

6. The goal is to make it malleable and then roll it out on a lightly floured parchment paper piece. Roll it out until you've reached a thickness of 0.5 cm, and cut 9cm circles out of the dough.

7. Oiled a cupcake tin with cooking spray, and line it with the 9 cm circles. Repeat until the cupcake tin is complete, and use another cupcake tin if there is dough left.

8. Add a spoonful of mincemeat in the center of every circle. Place it in the refrigerator to chill.

9. Roll out the remaining pastry 0.5cm thick, and transfer it to a separate baking sheet. Allow the muffin pan and baking sheet to chill in the refrigerator for 15 minutes.

10. Heat the oven to 350 degrees-Fahrenheit. Remove the pastry sheet from your fridge, and cut out 8cm circles.

11. Remove the mince pies from the refrigerator and place the circles on top of each one, covering the mixture. Drizzle the top of the mince pies with almond milk, and bake them in the oven for 30 minutes.

12. Remove from the oven, then cool down before serving them with an icing sugar pinch on top. Keep them in a sealable square container; refrigerate for 2 to 3 days. Serve chilled.

Nutrition:
Calories: 310
Carbohydrates: 37g
Protein: 4.2g

Fat: 14g

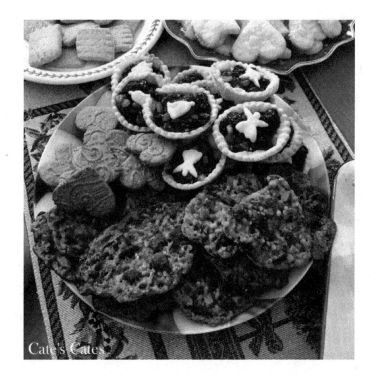

Strawberry Glow Sorbet

Preparation time: 15 minutes
Cooking time: 5 minutes
Servings: 4
Ingredients:

- 300ml of water
- 1 ¼ cups of caster sugar
- 3 ½ cups of strawberries (ripe)
- 1 lemon juice
- 1 tbsp of rose water

Directions:

1. Put the water plus sugar in a medium pan, and bring it to a boil for 1 minute.

2. Add strawberries to a blender, and pulse them until you've reached a smooth texture. Then, add the syrup from the sugar mixture to the blender with the juice of one lemon and rose water.

3. Transfer the strawberry mixture into an airtight container, and place it in the freezer for 1 to 2 hours. Freeze it for 6 to 7 days, or serve immediately, allowing it 15 minutes to soften before serving it.

Nutrition:
Calories: 240
Carbohydrates: 57g
Protein: 1.1g
Fat: 0.2g

Chocolate Cups

Preparation time: 15 minutes
Cooking time: 3 minutes
Servings: 4
Ingredients:

- 1 cup of cacao butter
- ½ cup of cacao powder
- ½ cup of cacao nibs
- 4 tbsps. of agave
- 1 tsp of water
- 1 tsp of vanilla extract
- ¼ tsp of Himalayan salt

Directions:

1. Add 12 cupcake liners to a mini muffin baking sheet, and set it aside. Add 1 tsp of water to a small pan over medium heat. Once boiling, place a bowl on top of the pan and ensure space between the bowl and water.

2. Add the cacao butter to the bowl for 2 minutes until it melts. Add the agave, and whisk the two ingredients to combine. Remove the bowl, and set it aside. Switch off the heat of the stove.

3. Add the cacao, salt, and vanilla extract to the bowl, and whisk the ingredients until combined. Add more agave for increased sweetness.

4. Pour the mixture into 12 mini cupcake liners. Add the cacao nibs on top of each, and transfer the muffin pan to the freezer. Freeze for 10 minutes or until set.

5. Place the mini cupcakes in an airtight container. Refrigerate for up to a week. Alternatively, store it in the freezer for up to 1 month.

Nutrition:
Calories: 160
Carbohydrates: 5.2g
Protein: 1.2g
Fat: 16.2g

Poached Caramel Peaches

Preparation time: 15 minutes
Cooking time: 0 minutes
Servings: 4
Ingredients:

- 2 cups of water (boiled)
- 1 cup of caster sugar
- 3 ripe peaches
- 1 lemon juice and zest
- 1/3 cup of blueberries
- 1 vanilla pod (cut in half, remove seeds)

Directions:

1. Bring a small pan to medium heat, and add the caster sugar to the pan, allowing it to caramelize. Swirl the sauce around in the pan without stirring it.
2. Once most of the sugar is caramelized, add 2 cups of boiled water to the pan, and stir the ingredients to combine, ensuring the sugar is dissolved.
3. Add lemon zest and the vanilla pod to the pan, cooking it for 5 minutes.
4. Cut the peaches in half, and remove the pits. Add the peaches to the syrup, and bring the ingredients to a simmer. Cook for 4 minutes, then switch off the heat.
5. Add the lemon juice to the pan and allow everything to cool down.
6. Divide the poached peaches into 4 glass mason jars, and add blueberries on top. Seal the jars, and refrigerate them for up to 3 days.

Nutrition:

Calories: 360
Carbohydrates: 94g
Protein: 1g
Fat: 1g

Coconut-Dipped Truffles

Preparation time: 15 minutes
Cooking time: 0 minutes
Servings: 4
Ingredients:

- 2 cups of coconut (shredded)
- ½ cup of macadamia nuts
- ¼ cup of cocoa butter (melted)
- 3 tbsp of stevia
- ½ tsp of vanilla extract
- ¼ tsp of Himalayan salt

Directions:

1. Add 1 ½ cups of coconut and the macadamia nuts to the food processor, and blend until you've reached a creamy paste consistency.
2. Add the melted cocoa butter, vanilla, salt, and stevia to the mixture, and mix them.
3. Add the mixture to a bowl. Place it in the refrigerator for at least 1 hour. Once done, add ½ cup of shredded coconut to the mixture, and mix it in.
4. Form the coconut truffles by spooning 1 tablespoon into a ball, rolling it with your hands, and placing them in a mason jar.
5. Place it in the refrigerator and store them for up to 1 week.

Nutrition:
Calories: 220
Carbohydrates: 7g
Protein: 1.6g
Fat: 21g

Cognac - Chocolate Roll

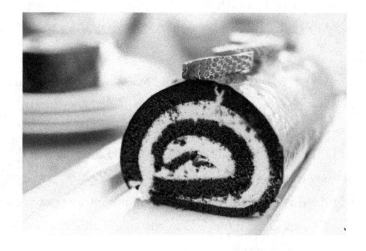

Preparation time: 15 minutes
Cooking time: 20 minutes
Servings: 10
Ingredients:

- 1 1/2 cups fresh butter
- 1 cup of powdered sugar
- 1/4 cup Cognac
- 4 Tbsp cocoa powder
- 1/2 lb. biscuits, plain crushed
- 1/2 cup of walnuts finely chopped

Directions:

1. Melt the butter in a microwave oven. In a saucepan, melt the butter and powdered sugar, cocoa powder, and cognac and stir well.
2. Add crushed biscuits and walnuts and stir well; allow the mixture to cool for 10 minutes. Spread the mixture onto foil or nonstick parchment paper and wrap it in a round shape.
3. Refrigerate for 3 – 4 hours; remove from fridge and slice. Freeze in a freezer-safe container for two months.

Nutrition:
Calories 463
Fat 35g
Carbohydrates 36.43g
Protein 3.42g

Cranberries and Hazelnuts Muffins

Preparation time: 15 minutes
Cooking time: 20 minutes
Servings: 16
Ingredients:

- 1/2 cup dried cranberries
- 1 cup boiling water
- 1 1/2 cup flour
- 1 Tbsp baking powder
- 5 ½ oz brown sugar
- 2 1/2 chopped hazelnuts
- 2 tsp dry ginger
- 1 tsp cinnamon powder
- 1/2 tsp nutmeg
- 3/4 cup sour milk
- 3/4 cup sunflower oil
- 1 large free-range egg, beaten

Coating:

- 2 Tbsp chopped hazelnuts
- 1 Tbsp brown sugar

Directions:

1. Put cranberries in a bowl and add the boiling water. Leave for 5-10 minutes and drain. Preheat the oven to 400 F/200 C.
2. Prepare and grease 16 baking muffin cups. Mix the flour with baking powder, sugar, hazelnuts, ginger, cinnamon, and nutmeg in a bowl.
3. In a separate bowl, beat the egg with sunflower oil and sour milk. Mix the liquid batter to the flour mixture. Add the cranberries and stir well until all ingredients are combined well.

4. Pour the mixture into prepared muffin cups. Sprinkle with hazelnuts and sugar and bake for about 20 minutes. Remove muffins from the oven, and let cool at room temperature.
5. Keep your muffins in sealed plastic bags for up to 3 days. Also, you can wrap muffins in freezer bags and freeze for up to 2 - 3 months.

Nutrition:
Calories 252
Fat 11.61g
Carbohydrates 35.72g
Protein 2.14g

Dark Knight Cake

Preparation time: 15 minutes
Cooking time: 25-30 minutes
Servings: 8
Ingredients:

- 1/4 cup cocoa powder unsweetened
- 2 cups flour, white, all-purpose
- 1/8 tsp salt
- 1/8 tsp baking powder
- 1/2 cup fresh butter, unsalted and melted
- 2 tbsp full-fat milk
- 1 1/2 tsp almond extract
- 2 tsp vanilla extract
- 1/4 cup brown sugar

Directions:

1. Preheat oven to 340F/165 degrees. Oiled a baking dish with a little butter. Stir the cocoa powder, flour, salt, and baking powder in a bowl.
2. In a separate bowl, whisk together melted butter, milk, almond and vanilla extract, and brown sugar until combined well.
3. Combine the flour mixture with the milk mixture and give a good stir. Put the batter in the prepared baking dish, and bake for 25 - 30 minutes.
4. Once ready, let cool at room temperature. Place in a container and keep refrigerated for up to one week.

Nutrition:
Calories 253
Fat 12.27g
Carbohydrates 32.47g

Protein 4.01g

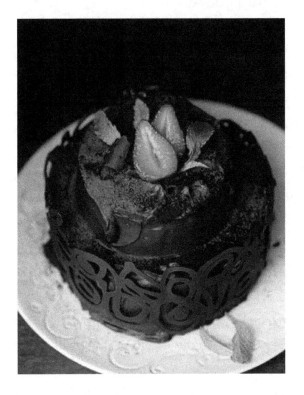

Oat - Flake Cookies with Raisins

Preparation time: 15 minutes
Cooking time: 8-10 minutes
Servings: 12
Ingredients:

- 1 1/2 cups flour for all uses
- 1 1/2 tsp baking powder
- 1 tsp cinnamon
- 1 pinch of salt
- 1 cup fresh butter unsalted
- 1 1/4 cups brown sugar
- 2 eggs, free-range
- 1 tsp vanilla powder
- 1 1/2 cups oat flakes
- 3/4 cup of raisins

Directions:

1. Soft at room temperature. Warm oven to 350 °F/175 ° C. Line a baking tray with parchment paper. Stir the flour with baking powder, cinnamon, and salt.
2. In a separate bowl, beat butter and sugar for 1 minute. Add the eggs and vanilla and continue to beat until all ingredients are combined well.
3. Add a flour mixture slowly; beat for a further 2 -3 minutes. Add the oat flakes and raisins and stir with a wooden spoon for one minute.
4. With a tablespoon, scoop a butter and place on the baking pan, leaving someplace between each cookie—Bake for about 8 to 10 minutes.

5. Remove your cookies, then let them cool completely. Put in a container, then keep refrigerated for one week, place muffins in a freezer-safe bag, and keep in a freezer.

Nutrition:
Calories 379
Fat 17g
Carbohydrates 54.37g
Protein 4.51g

Chocolate Cake

Preparation time: 15 minutes
Cooking time: 10 minutes
Servings: 8
Ingredients:

- 3/4 lb. chocolate covertures cut into small chunks
- 1 1/2 cups Nutella chocolate-hazelnut spread
- 1 cup fresh butter

Directions:

1. Grease a square tray and set aside. In a small saucepan, heat the covertures along with Nutella and butter over low heat.

2. Stir until the ingredients melt and combined well; stir frequently. Pour the mixture on the prepared tray, and straighten the surface with the back of a spoon. Refrigerate the cake overnight.

3. Remove the cake from the refrigerator, cut it into square pieces. Put it with a cover in the refrigerator for one week. Store cake in a freezer-safe bag and keep in a freezer for 3 months.

Nutrition:
Calories 449
Fat 39.31g
Carbohydrates 22.31g
Protein 2.84g

Semolina Cake with Syrup

Preparation time: 15 minutes
Cooking time: 1 hour & 21 minutes
Servings: 14
Ingredients:

- 1 1/2 cup coarse semolina
- 1 1/2 cup fine semolina
- 1 1/2 cup sugar
- 2 1/2 cups of yogurt
- 2 tsp of baking powder
- 1 tsp pure vanilla extract

For the syrup:

- 1 1/2 cup water
- 2 1/2 cup brown sugar (or stevia sweetener)

Directions:

1. Preheat oven to 360 F/180 C. Grease a rectangular baking pan with a little oil and set aside. Combine all ingredients in a mixing bowl; with an electric mixer, beat until compact mixture is achieved.

2. Pour the batter into a prepared baking pan—Bake for 1 hour and 15 minutes. Remove the cake, then cut diagonally while it's still hot.

3. Cook water and sugar over medium heat for 5 - 6 minutes or until sugar is completely dissolved and you get a thick syrup. Pour hot syrup over the cake.

4. Let cool at room temperature; cover with foil, and keep refrigerated. Store cake in a freezer-safe container, and keep in a freezer.

Nutrition:
Calories 389
Fat 1g
Carbohydrates 89g
Protein 6g

Avocado Chocolate Mousse

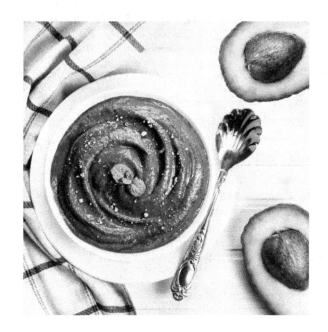

Preparation time: 15 minutes
Cooking time: 0 minutes
Servings: 8
Ingredients:

- 2 large ripe avocados
- 4 tablespoons maple syrup or honey
- 4 tablespoons almond milk
- 8 tablespoons cocoa powder
- 20 drops of liquid stevia/2 tablespoons of syrup or honey
- Cacao nibs or coconut flakes or strawberries, optional

Directions:

1. Mix all the ingredients in a blender until it becomes smooth and creamy. Allow it to freeze before serving.
2. Serve it in a bowl or wine glass, garnished with desired toppings. It can be store in the refrigerator for 2-3 days.

Nutrition:
Calories: 201
Carbs: 20g
Fat: 15g
Protein: 45g

Chocolate Chia Pudding

Preparation time: 15 minutes
Cooking time: 0 minutes
Servings: 8
Ingredients:

- 2 Tablespoons chia seeds
- 6 tablespoons milk
- Coconut flakes, cacao nibs or berries, optional
- 2 Tablespoons cocoa powder
- 20 drops of liquid stevia or 2 or more tablespoons of honey

Directions:

1. Take a container or a jar and add all the ingredients to it. Now using a fork, whisk until the chia seeds get immersed in the liquid properly.
2. Taste to make sure the mixture's sweetness is to your liking, or add more according to your taste buds.
3. Keep it overnight in the fridge or for a minimum of 12 hours for the best results. Serve when required. It can last for 2-3 days in the refrigerator.

Nutrition:
Calories: 80
Carbs: 14g
Fat: 3g
Protein: 2g

Vegan Coconut Oil Chocolates

Preparation time: 15 minutes
Cooking time: 0 minutes
Servings: 8
Ingredients:

- ¼cup melted coconut oil
- 1 tablespoon mesquite powder
- 1/8 cup toasted almonds
- 1/8 cup raw cacao powder
- 1 tablespoon maple syrup
- 1/8 cup shredded or flaked coconut

Directions:

1. Add coconut oil, cacao powder, mesquite powder, and maple syrup in a bowl and incorporate well until combined.
2. Take half of the number of almonds and coconut and add to this mixture and fold. The rest of the almonds and coconut can be used for garnishing.
3. Take 6-8 small cupcake liners and place them in a baking pan. Add mixture to these cupcake liners and garnish with the rest of the almonds and coconuts.
4. Cool it in a refrigerator for around 2 hours before serving. It can be stored in the fridge for up to a week and served as and when required.

Nutrition:
Calories: 60
Carbs: 3g
Fat: 5g
Protein: 0g

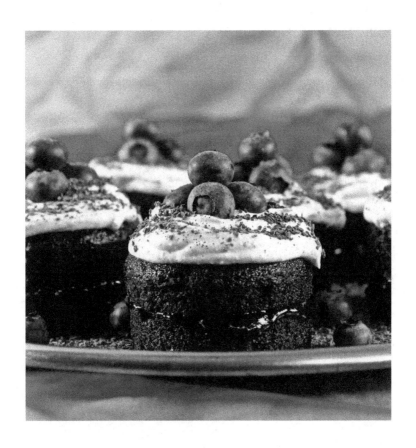

Fresh Berries with Yogurt and Chocolate

Preparation time: 15 minutes
Cooking time: 0 minutes
Servings: 5
Ingredients:

- 1 basket of fresh strawberries
- 1 basket of fresh raspberries
- 4-ounce dark chocolate, melted in a double boiler
- 16-ounce low-fat vanilla yogurt

Directions:

1. Mix berries in a large bowl. Add yogurt and fold gently. Serve berries along with yogurt in individual bowls. Drizzle melted chocolate over it and serve.

Nutrition:
Calories: 231
Carbs: 0g
Fat: 0g
Protein: 15g

Chocolate Peanut Butter Ice Cream

Preparation time: 15 minutes
Cooking time: 0 minutes
Servings: 8
Ingredients:

- 4 big bananas, frozen and sliced
- 4 tablespoons creamy natural peanut butter
- ½teaspoon cinnamon
- 4 tablespoons cocoa powder
- 1 teaspoon vanilla
- 1-2 pinches of salt

Directions:

1. Add all the fixings to a food processor and pulse slowly, around 15 seconds at a time, until smooth and creamy. It can be frozen in an airtight container for up to 5 days or served immediately.

Nutrition:
Calories: 250
Carbs: 24g
Fat: 16g
Protein: 5g

Triple Coconut Cream Pie

Preparation time: 15 minutes
Cooking time: 15 minutes
Servings: 8
Ingredients:
For the Custard:

- 4 eggs
- 1 cup of sugar
- 1 cup skim milk
- ½teaspoon vanilla extract
- ½cup flour
- 1-2 pinches of salt
- 2-13.5 ounce can of light coconut milk

For the Coconut Whipped Cream:

- 2-13.5 ounce can of coconut milk, refrigerated
- 4 tablespoons confectioner's sugar
- 1 teaspoon vanilla extract For the Pie:
- 2 prebaked pie crust
- 6 tablespoons toasted coconut

Directions:
To Prepare Custard:

1. Add eggs, flour, sugar, and salt in a big bowl. Wisk together and set aside. Take a big saucepan to add skim milk and coconut milk. Cook on low until it bubbles alongside the pan.

2. Remove from heat. Pour milk into the mixture whisking all the while quickly. Now pour this mixture back into the saucepan and place it over low heat. Let it simmer for about 10-12 minutes until thick and bubbly.

3. Once the mixture thickens, take it off from the heat and transfer it to a heatproof bowl. Freeze it until the custard is room temperature. Add vanilla extract.

To Prepare the Coconut Whipped Cream:

4. Spoon out the top cream portion of the refrigerated coconut cream into a mixer. Wisk on high for around 3-4 minutes until stiff peaks are formed. Add vanilla and confectioner's sugar.

To assemble the Pie:

5. Now pour the cooled custard into the crust. Garnish with whipped cream and toasted coconut. Cover with cling film and freeze for around 6 hours until the custard is chilled.

Nutrition:
Calories: 330
Carbs: 39g
Fat: 18g
Protein: 2g

Carrot Cake Energy Bites

Preparation time: 15 minutes
Cooking time: 0 minutes
Servings: 8
Ingredients:

- ½cup walnuts
- 12 Medjool dates, pitted
- ½cup finely shredded coconut + extra to top
- 1 cup carrots, finely grated + extra to top
- ¼teaspoon sea salt
- 1 teaspoon ground nutmeg

Directions:

1. Add dates, ½ cup carrots, coconut, salt, and nutmeg into a food processor and pulse until smooth. Add remaining carrots and walnuts and pulse until you get a coarse texture with the nuts visible.
2. Transfer into a bowl. Divide and shape into 20 balls. Roll each in extra shredded coconut and place on a lined baking sheet. Garnish with carrots and serve.
3. Refrigerate the balls until ready to serve. Keep the unused ones refrigerated. It can last for 4-5 days when refrigerated.

Nutrition:
Calories: 73
Carbs: 8g
Fat: 4g
Protein: 2g

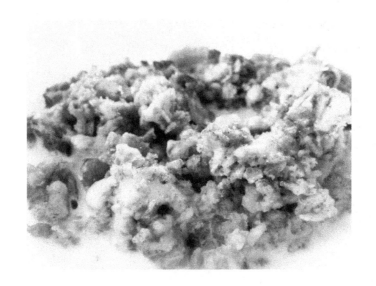

Vanilla Coconut and Chia Seed Pudding

Preparation time: 15 minutes
Cooking time: 0 minutes
Servings: 8
Ingredients:

- ½ cup shredded, unsweetened coconut
- ½ cup chia seeds
- 1 ½ cups full fat coconut milk
- 1 cup of coconut water
- 2 teaspoons pure vanilla extract
- ½ teaspoon salt
- 1 cup fresh raspberries to serve

Directions:

1. Mix all the fixings except raspberries in a bowl. Pour into serving bowls and refrigerate until use. Serve with fresh raspberries.

Nutrition:
Calories: 265
Carbs: 12g
Fat: 11g
Protein: 19g

Vanilla Puffed Quinoa Peanut Butter Balls

Preparation time: 15 minutes
Cooking time: 10 minutes
Servings: 8
Ingredients:

- 2 cups puffed quinoa
- 1 cup peanut butter
- ½ cup agave nectar or honey or pure maple syrup
- 2 tablespoons peanuts, roasted, crushed
- 2 teaspoons vanilla extract
- Dark chocolate, melted for dipping (optional)

Directions:

1. Mix in a heatproof bowl, peanut butter, agave, and vanilla. Place the bowl in a double boiler until the ingredients are softened and smooth flowing. Whisk as it is softening.
2. Remove from heat and add puffed quinoa. Mix well and refrigerate for 15-20 minutes.
3. Remove from the refrigerator and divide the mixture into 12-15 equal portions and shape into small balls. Dip into dark chocolate if desired. Refrigerate until set. It can store for a week.

Nutrition:
Calories: 82
Carbs: 12g
Fat: 4g
Protein: 0g

Walnut Fruit Cookies

Preparation time: 15 minutes
Cooking time: 0 minutes
Servings: 8
Ingredients:

- ½ cup natural almond butter/any other nut butter of your choice
- 8 scoops vanilla or chocolate protein powder
- 2 tablespoons ground flaxseeds
- 4 cups rolled oats
- 2 teaspoons cocoa powder, unsweetened
- 1 cup of water
- ¼ cup raisins
- 2 tablespoons dried cranberries
- 2 tablespoons walnuts, chopped

Directions:

1. Mix all the fixings in a bowl to form a dough-like consistency. Shape into cookies and place on a dish that is lined with parchment paper. Refrigerate until use. It can last for a week.

Nutrition:
Calories: 110
Carbs: 19g
Fat: 4g
Protein: 1g

Coconut Berries Ice Cream

Preparation time: 15 minutes
Cooking time: 0 minutes
Servings: 5
Ingredients:

- 2 cups of coconut milk
- ½ pound frozen strawberries /blueberries, unsweetened
- Stevia or sugar to taste
- ¼ tablespoon lemon juice or to taste

Directions:

1. Place all fixings in the food processor and blend until smooth. Transfer into a freezer-safe container. Freeze until firm.
2. Alternately transfer the blended mixture into an ice cream maker and follow the manufacturer's instructions to freeze.
3. Remove from the freezer 30 minutes before serving. Scoop and serve in dessert bowls.

Nutrition:
Calories: 116
Carbs: 11g
Fat: 74g
Protein: 1g

Orange Chia Seeds Parfait

Preparation time: 15 minutes
Cooking time: 0 minutes
Servings: 5
Ingredients:

- ½ cups orange juice
- ¼ cup chia seeds
- 2 tablespoons agave nectar/maple syrup or sweetener of your choice
- 1 banana, sliced
- 1 cup fresh berries of your choice

Directions:

1. Pour orange juice into a bowl. Add chia seeds. Stir well. Cover and keep it aside for 10 minutes. Stir in between. If the chia seeds have not absorbed all the orange juice, then blend with a stick blender.
2. Divide the chia seeds into 2 glasses. Layer alternately with berries and bananas. Chill and serve later. It can store for 2 days.

Nutrition:
Calories: 100
Carbs: 21g
Fat: 1g
Protein: 2g

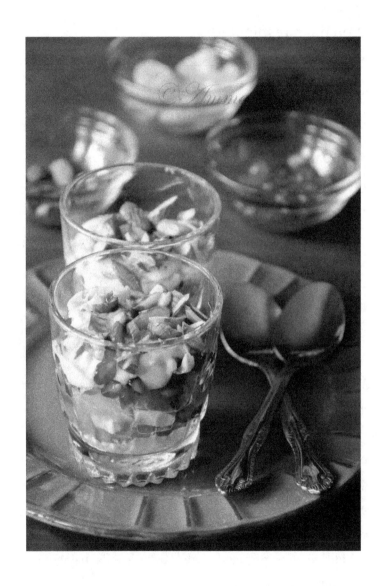

Vanilla Almond Banana Muffins and Peanut Butter

Preparation time: 15 minutes
Cooking time: 20 minutes
Servings: 5
Ingredients:

- 1+1/4 teaspoon baking powder
- 1+1/2 cup (3 large) bananas, mashed overripe
- 1/3 cup smooth/creamy peanut butter, organic, unsalted
- 1/2 teaspoon cinnamon
- 1/2 teaspoon baking soda
- 1/2 cup unsweetened applesauce
- 1/2 cup unsweetened almond milk/your preferred milk
- 1 teaspoon pure vanilla extract
- 1 cup quick oats
- 1 cup protein powder, vanilla

Swirl:

- 3 tablespoon creamy peanut butter, organic, unsalted, and divided

Directions:

1. Preheat oven to375F. Grease a nonstick (high-quality) 12-muffin tin thoroughly with cooking spray. Set aside.
2. Whisk the milk, peanut butter, mashed bananas, applesauce, and the vanilla extract in a large mixing bowl, w.
3. Add in the oats, protein powder, baking soda, baking powder, and cinnamon. Stir gently until combined. The batter will be thick.

4. Fill each tin with the batter about 2/3 full—Bake for 20 minutes. Remove the tins from the oven. Let it cool in the tin within 45 minutes, and then transfer to a cooling rack.
5. Place in an airtight container. Store in a cool, dry place for up to 3 days or refrigerate for up to 5 to 6 days.

Nutrition:
Calories: 149
Carbs: 25g
Fat: 4g
Protein: 5g

Maple Syrup Coconut Custard

Preparation time: 15 minutes
Cooking time: 45-50 minutes
Servings: 5
Ingredients:

- 5 egg yolks
- 13 1/2 fluid ounces coconut milk, canned
- 1/4 cups coconut flour
- 1/4 cups arrowroot powder
- 1/2 teaspoons sea salt
- 1/2 teaspoons cardamom, ground
- 1 tablespoon maple syrup
- 1 cup coconut flakes, toasted
- 1 cup applesauce
- 1 1/2 cups coconut cream

For serving:

- 1/2 cups blackberries
- 1/2 cups blueberries

Directions:

1. In a bowl, whisk coconut milk, coconut cream, egg yolks, applesauce, and maple syrup. Combine the arrowroot powder, coconut flour, cardamom, and sea salt in another bowl.
2. Mix the dry fixings into the wet fixings until smooth. Put the mix into a 9x13 baking dish. Bake at 350F for about 45 to 50 minutes or until set.
3. The custard will set as it cooks. Sprinkle the top of the custard with toasted coconut flakes and top with berries.

4. Allow the custard to cool thoroughly. Cut the custard into 8 pieces of 10-ounce cups. Sprinkle top with toasted coconut flakes. Cover with plastic wrap and freeze.
5. When serving, it can be served cool or microwave for about 20 to 30 minutes to warm. Top with berries. Enjoy.

Nutrition:
Calories: 300
Carbs: 42g
Fat: 0g
Protein: 4g

Honey-Broiled Nectarines

Preparation time: 15 minutes
Cooking time: 6-8 minutes
Servings: 5
Ingredients:

- 2 large nectarines, pitted, halved
- 1 tablespoon lemon juice
- 3 tablespoons honey

Directions:

1. Place the nectarine halves with its cut side facing up in a baking dish. Mix honey plus lemon juice in a bowl.
2. Brush this mixture over the nectarines. Broil in a preheated broiler for 6-8 minutes. Serve warm. To store, place in an airtight container and refrigerate until use.

Nutrition:
Calories: 44
Carbs: 11g
Fat: 0g
Protein: 1g

Buttermilk Almond Vanilla Oat Waffles

Preparation time: 15 minutes
Cooking time: 4-5 minutes
Servings: 5
Ingredients:

- 2/3 cup whole-wheat flour
- 2/3 cup almond flour
- 2 teaspoons vanilla extract
- 2 large eggs, lightly beaten
- 2 cups buttermilk
- 1/4 teaspoon salt
- 1/4 cup toasted wheat germ/cornmeal
- 1/4 cup brown sugar
- 1/2 teaspoon baking soda
- 1/2 cup rolled oats, old-fashioned
- 1 teaspoon ground cinnamon
- 1 tablespoon canola oil
- 1 1/2 teaspoons baking powder

Directions:

1. In a medium-sized bowl, mix the buttermilk with the oats; let stand for 15 minutes. Inside a large bowl, whisk the flours with the wheat germ/cornmeal, baking soda, baking powder, cinnamon, and salt.
2. Stir the eggs, oil, brown sugar, and vanilla into the oat mix. Add the wet ingredients into the dry ingredients; with a rubber spatula, mix until just moistened.
3. Oiled a waffle iron with cooking spray and preheat. Spoon just enough batter to cover 3/4 of the waffle iron surface, about 2/3 cup for an 8x8 waffle iron.

---

4. Cook for about 4-5 minutes or till the waffle is golden brown and crisp. Repeat the process with the remaining batter.

5. Individually wrap the waffles with plastic wrap; refrigerate for up 2 days or freeze for up to 1 month. When ready to serve, just reheat in a toaster oven or toaster. For long-term freezing, wrap the loaf or slices or muffins with plastic wrap and then with foil.

Nutrition:
Calories: 260
Carbs: 29g
Fat: 11g
Protein: 12g

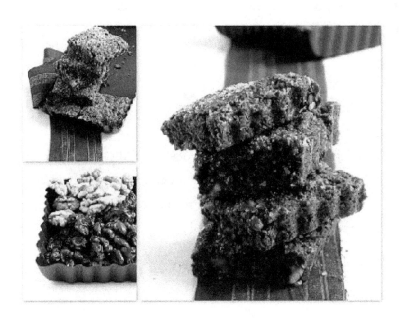

Vanilla Cocoa Bananas Peanut Butter Ice Cream

Preparation time: 15 minutes
Cooking time: 0 minutes
Servings: 5
Ingredients:

- 4 big bananas, frozen and sliced
- 4 tablespoons creamy natural peanut butter
- ½teaspoon cinnamon
- 4 tablespoons cocoa powder
- 1 teaspoon vanilla
- 1-2 pinches of salt

Directions:

1. Add all the fixings to a food processor and pulse slowly, around 15 seconds at a time, until smooth and creamy. It can be frozen in an airtight container for up to 5 days or served immediately.

Nutrition:
Calories: 120
Carbs: 16g
Fat: 5g
Protein: 4g

Coconut Whipped Cream Pie

Preparation time: 15 minutes
Cooking time: 10-12 minutes
Servings: 5
Ingredients:
For the Custard:

- 4 eggs
- 1 cup of sugar
- 1 cup skim milk
- ½teaspoon vanilla extract
- ½cup flour
- 1-2 pinches of salt
- 2-13.5 ounce can of light coconut milk

For the Coconut Whipped Cream:

- 2-13.5 ounce can of coconut milk, refrigerated
- 4tablespoons confectioner's sugar
- 1 teaspoon vanilla extract
- For the Pie:
- 2 prebaked pie crust
- 6 tablespoons toasted coconut

Directions:
To Prepare Custard:

1. Add eggs, flour, sugar, and salt in a big bowl. Wisk together and set aside. Take a big saucepan to add skim milk and coconut milk.
2. Cook on low until it bubbles along the side of the pan. Remove from heat. Pour milk into the mixture whisking all the while quickly.

3. Now pour this mixture back into the saucepan and place it over low heat. Let it simmer for about 10-12 minutes until thick and bubbly.

4. Once the mixture thickens, take it off from the heat and transfer it to a heatproof bowl. Freeze it until the custard is room temperature. Add vanilla extract.

For the Coconut Whipped Cream:

5. Spoon out the top cream portion of the refrigerated coconut cream into a mixer. Wisk on high for around 3-4 minutes until stiff peaks are formed. Add vanilla and confectioner's sugar.

To Assemble the Pie:

6. Now pour the cooled custard into the crust. Garnish with whipped cream and toasted coconut. Cover with cling film and freeze for around 6 hours until the custard is chilled.

Nutrition:
Calories: 230
Carbs: 18g
Fat: 10g
Protein: 1g

Carrot Nutmeg Cake

Preparation time: 15 minutes
Cooking time: 0 minutes
Servings: 5
Ingredients:

- ½cup walnuts
- 12 Medjool dates, pitted
- ½cup finely shredded coconut + extra to top
- 1 cup carrots, finely grated + extra to top
- ¼teaspoon sea salt
- 1 teaspoon ground nutmeg

Directions:

1. Add dates, ½ cup carrots, coconut, salt, and nutmeg into a food processor and pulse until smooth. Add remaining carrots and walnuts and pulse until you get a coarse texture with the nuts visible.
2. Transfer into a bowl. Divide and shape into 20 balls. Roll each in extra shredded coconut and place on a lined baking sheet. Garnish with carrots and serve.
3. Refrigerate the balls until ready to serve. Keep the unused ones refrigerated. It can last for 4-5 days when refrigerated.

Nutrition:
Calories: 94
Carbs: 10g
Fat: 1g
Protein: 10g

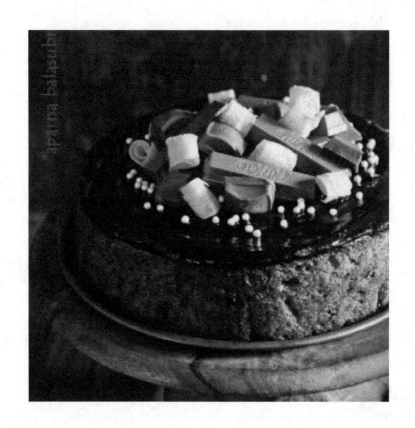

Bananas Berries Fruit Fudgy

Preparation time: 15 minutes
Cooking time: 0 minutes
Servings: 5
Ingredients:

- Chocolate chips (2 tbsp., less sweetened)
- Bananas (2, large-sized, peeled and cut into small pieces)
- Strawberries (8, large sized)
- Peanuts (1/4 cups, chopped and unsalted)

Directions:

1. Let the chocolate chips melt in a small bowl in a microwave oven on high heat for about 10 seconds. Periodically repeat the heating until the chips melt completely. Keep stirring the chips.
2. Now in a small tray, put waxed paper and cover the tray with it. Add the melted chocolate to the fruit that is placed on the paper.
3. Then add nuts to the fruits and cover it and refrigerate the whole thing for about 20 minutes or 10 minutes; it depends upon when the chocolate hardens itself. After taking it out, serve immediately.

Nutrition:
Calories: 133
Carbs: 34g
Fat: 0g
Protein: 1g

30-Day Meal Plan

Day	Breakfast	Lunch	Snack	Dinner	Dessert
1	Spinach-Berry Smoothie Pack	Stuffed Bell Peppers	Banana Nut Muffins	Crispy Baked Fish Sticks	Lemon Bars
2	Morning Sunshine Smoothie Pack	Vegetarian Buddha Bowl	Hummus Deviled Eggs	Mexican Chicken and Veggie Brochettes with Salsa Dip	Almond Butter Cheesecake
3	Blackberry Bran Muffins	Southwestern Chicken Wraps	Chocolate Zucchini Muffins	Chinese Orange Chicken with Broccoli Basmati	Coconut Cookie Dough
4	Pear-Pumpkin Seed Muffins	Snapper En Papillote	Apple-Cinnamon Greek Yogurt Parfait	Pressed Caesar Tuna Melts	Chocolate Tart
5	Pumpkin Breakfast Blondies	Feta Turkey Burgers	Edamame Hummus with Jicama Sticks	Tahini Tuna Salad Stacks	Strawberry Cheesecake
6	Blueberry-Zucchini Waffles	Heathy Shepherd's Pie	PB and Jelly Greek Yogurt Jars	Polenta with Texas Turkey Ragu	Flourless Chocolate Cookies

7	Cranberry-Pistachio Granola with Yogurt	Spiced Salmon with Roasted Broccoli and Cauliflower	Honey and Orange Corn Muffins	Sloppy Joe-Smothered Sweet Potato Fries	Lemon Cheesecake Mousse
8	Quinoa and Berries Breakfast Bowl	Greek Grilled Chicken Salad	Corn and Bean Salsa with Chips	Mushroom Veggie Burgers	Cashew Butter Mousse
9	Tropical Parfait	Deconstructed Taco Bowls	Turkey Roll-Ups	Quinoa Tabbouleh with Hummus	Mint Chocolate Brownies
10	Make-Ahead Cottage Cheese and Fruit Bowl	Turkey-Apple-Walnut Kale Salad	Cucumber Smoked Salmon Rolls	Spicy Sichuan Beef with Mixed Vegetables	Pumpkin Pie Bites
11	Peanut Butter-Banana Oatmeal	Simple Lentil Salad	Baked Jalapeno Poppers	Chicken Pasta with Creamy Vodka Sauce	Chocolate Pudding
12	Banana-Strawberry Oatmeal Cups	Vietnamese Beef Noodle Bowl	Dried Fruit and Nut Dark Chocolate Bark	Veggie Spaghetti Lo Mein	Cinnamon Bites
13	Triple Berry Oatmeal-Almond Bake	Chicken Tortilla Soup	Peanut Butter Banana Energy Cookies	Turmeric-Pistachio Pilaf with Spicy Italian Sausage	Pistachio Fudge

14	Veggie Delight Breakfast Egg Casserole	Best Bunless Burgers	Apricot-Orange Oat Bites	Pork Tenderloin with Mediterranean Quinoa Salad	Vanilla Mascarpone Parfait
15	Egg and Spinach Stuffed Peppers	Broccoli Salad	Chocolate Energy Balls	Spinach Pasta Fazool	Pumpkin Spice Pudding
16	Pineapple Ginger Parfait	Curried Red Lentil Soup	No-Bake Maple Cinnamon Bars	Zesty Lentil Zuppa Toscana	Sunflower Butter Chocolate Bars
17	Apple Nut Butter Quesadilla	Grilled Mediterranean Chicken Kabobs	Honey Ricotta with Strawberries	Pan-Seared Eggplant Medallions with Balsamic Reduction	Peanut Butter Cookies
18	Chocolate Cherry Oatmeal Cups	Flank Steak with Pan-Seared Brussels Sprouts	Homemade Trail Mix	Oven Roasted Garlic Chicken Thighs	Chocolate Coconut Clusters
19	Blueberry Fool Overnight Oatmeal Oats	Buffalo Chicken Salad	Crudité with Herbed Yogurt Dip	Roasted Carrot Ginger Bisque	Peanut Butter Fudge
20	Zucchini Cheddar Scones	Chicken Cobb Salad	Chili-Roasted Chickpeas	Garlic Lentil Bowls	Snickerdoodle Cupcakes

21	Good Morning Sweet Potato Jacket	Chicken Tikka Masala	Thyme-Roasted Almonds	Balsamic Chicken with Summer Vegetables	Pineapple Spice Sorbet
22	Strawberry Balsamic French Toast Bake	Cashew Chicken and Peppers	Cinnamon Cocoa Popcorn	Caprese Stuffed Chicken	Cherry Almond Brownies
23	Pumpkin Pancakes	Sweet Potato Chicken Nuggets and Parsnip Fries	Fruit Salad with Mint	Mediterranean Quinoa Bake	Raspberry Chia Pudding
24	Mushroom Asparagus Quiche with Quinoa Crust	Chicken, Spinach, and Tomatoes in Cream Sauce	Mason Jar Key Lime Parfaits	Honey Garlic Chicken Thighs	Sweet Tiffin
25	Italian Sausage Breakfast Bake	Skillet Chicken with Tomatoes and Shallots	Sriracha Hummus	Spaghetti Squash and Meatballs	Banana Peanut Butter Muffins
26	Bircher Muesli with Apple and Cinnamon	Carnitas Burrito Bowls	Rosemary Beet Chips	Lemon Salmon with White Beans	Vegan Mince Pies

27	Prepped Fruit Salad with Lemon and Honey	Zoodles with Meatballs and Pesto Sauce	Sriracha-Lime Kale Chips	Grilled Chicken with Homemade Tzatziki	Strawberry Glow Sorbet
28	Berry, Yogurt and Chia Pots	Korean-Style Beef and Broccoli Bowl	Avocado Chips	Cauliflower Prawn Casserole	Chocolate Cups
29	Salmon and Egg Muffins	Meatloaf and Mashed Cauliflower	Ant on a Log	Cheesy Tuna Pate	Poached Caramel Peaches
30	Green Smoothie Freezer Packets	Short Rib and Root Veggie Stew	Rice Cake Topped with Avocado	Cod Fritters	Coconut-Dipped Truffles

Conclusion

Preparing meals at a go might seem difficult initially, especially if you are completely a beginner to the idea of controlling portion sizes, working on meal prep meals, or cooking with healthy ingredients. But with regular practice and proper planning, you will soon get to know that it can be beneficial to get back to clean eating track mode.

Meal prepping is by no means something that you can do in a day. Just the way that you can't eat a big meal on an empty stomach. It usually takes several days of eating clean and healthy to get back into the routine of eating the right foods. If you believe in the saying that we are what we eat, you probably already know that prepping your meals each week is an excellent way to improve your health and eliminate eating out during the week. Plus, it allows you to expand your skills and abilities. It enables you to do a lot more with a lot less.

This Meal Prep Cookbook provided you with recipes that can help you create healthy and delicious food daily. They help you to maintain a proper and healthy eating plan. The prepping meal process also allows you to create a schedule for the week for healthy eating. Together with exercise, this can provide you with some of the best habits that can be helpful in your journey to lead a better and healthier life.

Meal prepping is mostly done on weekends. It let you spend more time with your loved ones. It helps you to look better, feel more energized, and have a more positive outlook during the week. It helps to manage your stress level as well.

Another reason for preparing meals during the weekend is that fresh foods tend to be drenched in the spices you use for each recipe. It is much easier to work with raw foods, especially if you are not used to the spices used to prepare them. It helps you to prepare the dish and plan your week ahead. You can also store the food for a later date.

If you are new to the journey of meal prepping and you have never done this type of cooking before, it is essential to do some research before starting. This cookbook helps you learn how meal prepping works, how it can help you, and how to do it properly. There are tons of things that are needed to keep in mind when you are prepping the meals. When you are cooking, you should always serve healthy food. It will ensure that you will consume food that is full of life-enhancing nutrients. Foods such as animal proteins (meat) provide all the energy, minerals, and vitamins you need. However, if these are not included in your meal, it can adversely affect your body.

The most common and helpful meal prep recipes contain healthy ingredients that are perfect for your health. Many recipes in this book use salads with beans and chickpeas, chicken, eggs, fish, oats, and creamy soups. Some recipes combine a bit of all of these and create the perfect meal for you to consume.

Cooking with veggies and ingredients is considered healthy cooking. It means that you need to have a healthy cookbook that contains recipes that are easy to prepare and healthy for you to consume. You will also need to select the ingredients that you want to include in your meals. The only way to naturally prepare food is to use the best kitchenware, accessories, and best-fit accessories. All these methods will help you to prepare food with convenience and ease.

We hope that you will decide to meal prep more often. You will be stun at how easy it is and how many healthy meals and snacks you can make. You are no longer need to worry about being in the grocery store for hours trying to find a good meal or snack. Preparing your meals in advance allows and help you to stay away from unhealthy foods for the week and keep them off for more effective weight control.

Meal prepping might be useful for maintaining habits. Along with the proper diet and regular exercise, meal prepping has the potential to be a life-saving habit.

I hope you have learned something!

CPSIA information can be obtained
at www.ICGtesting.com
Printed in the USA
BVHW092053190421
605311BV00002B/63

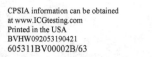